Also available

Puzzling Out... Anaesthesia

Puzzling Out... General Medicine Part 1

GW00793187

Coming in Spring 2005

Puzzling Out...Clinical Signs & Symptoms

Puzzling Out...General Medicine Part 2

Puzzling Out...Obstetrics & Gynaecology

Puzzling Out...Orthopaedics

Published by Remedica

32–38 Osnaburgh Street, London, NW1 3ND, UK

20 N Wacker Drive, Suite 1642, Chicago, IL, USA

info@remedicabooks.com

www.remedicabooks.com

Tel: +44 20 7388 7677

Fax: +44 20 7388 7678

Publisher: Andrew Ward

In-house editor: Cath Harris

British Library Cataloguing-in-Publication Data

A catalogue record for this book is available from the British Library.

INTRODUCTION

So, then. What's all this about? Puzzle books? To learn medicine from? That can't be right. Medicine is far too serious for that… Or is it?

These books were conceived by consultants with many years' experience of teaching medical students, who noticed a few things. Firstly, students are poorer than ever. They can't afford £25 for a textbook on each new topic. Secondly, there is a limit to how much anyone can 'take in' at one sitting. Medical knowledge might be better delivered in 'bite-sized pieces'. Thirdly, studying a book after a long day on the wards can be desperately dull. This should not be the case!

Following the success of a puzzle book for the MRCP exam (*My First MRCP Book*, Remedica, 2004) come these texts. And who has written them? Young doctors, and even final-year medical students – all right on the ball with what you need to know. They offer you all the key knowledge that you need to pass finals. No more, no less. This isn't to say that these books are exhaustive: you will learn more from ward teaching, lectures, and other books. The books are coat-hangers, if you will, upon which to hang other learning.

So there you have it! Read. Learn. Digest. But ultimately, enjoy. Medicine is, after all, the best profession in the world.

How to use these books

In some cases, these books are a pot pourri of information into which you can dip. This is deliberate: after all, it is the way patients present!

In other cases a whole subject is covered in one book. Here, you might want to start at one end and work your way through. However, you might also wish to 'dip in', perhaps looking up a topic you've heard about in a clinic that day. If so, feel free!

In every case, you will find the puzzle on one page, with the answer on the reverse. Turn the book upside down and you will find a short résumé of that subject. Remember – these are cheap books, so feel free to augment the text with notes and scrawls. When exam time looms, we suggest that you turn the book upside down, and read only the 'text' pages. In this way, you will find that you have a complete text (and note) book at your fingertips!

We wish you luck.

Jagdeep K Rai, Neil Goldsack, Hugh Montgomery

CONTENTS

PUZZLE I   ARTHRITIS

Arthritis means inflammation of the joints. There are a variety of causes, which can be remembered in a number of different ways. One is to use a standard surgical sieve – TIE HIM IN. Using this approach, can you connect the headings with the causes of arthritis? Some causes come under more than one heading…

Headings	Causes
Traumatic	Acromegaly
Infective	Rheumatic fever
Endocrine	Rheumatoid arthritis
Haematological	Crystal arthropathies
Immune/idiopathic	SLE
Metabolic	Enteropathic arthritis
Iatrogenic	Reiter's syndrome
Neoplastic	Septic arthritis
	Haemarthrosis
	TB
	Ankylosing spondylitis
	Osteoarthritis
	Gout
	Sickle cell crisis
	Scleroderma

PUZZLE I — ARTHRITIS

Traumatic
Haemarthrosis • Osteoarthritis

Infective
Pyogenic arthritis • Reiter's syndrome • Rheumatic fever • TB

Endocrine
Acromegaly

Haematological
Gout • Haemarthrosis • Sickle cell crisis

Immune/idiopathic
Ankylosing spondylitis • Enteropathic arthritis • Reiter's syndrome • Rheumatic fever • Rheumatoid arthritis • Scleroderma • SLE

Metabolic
Crystal arthropathies (gout)

Iatrogenic
Gout, SLE

Neoplastic
Crystal arthropathies (gout)

The causes of arthritis can be remembered with the mnemonic TIE HIM IN:

Traumatic • **I**nfective • **E**ndocrine • **H**aematological • **I**mmune/Idiopathic • **M**etabolic • **I**atrogenic • **N**eoplastic

Traumatic
- Haemarthrosis is the presence of blood in the joint. The joint becomes acutely swollen and painful, often to the point of greatly restricted movement. The nature of the underlying joint injury should be assessed. The joint may need draining surgically, so consult your surgical orthopaedic colleagues early. Haemarthrosis is a common complication in patients with haemophilia and may occur with only minor trauma.
- Recurrent 'wear and tear' may contribute to the development of osteoarthritis. Osteoarthritis is a common long-term sequelae of a fracture.

Infective
Infection may directly involve the joint:
- Septic arthritis (see Puzzle 27) is where bacteria grow in the joint itself. This is an EMERGENCY – the joint may need immediate drainage/surgical intervention, so call for help at once.
- TB may chronically involve the joints.

Alternatively, infection may trigger an auto-immune attack on the joints:
- TB can do this, as well as directly affecting the joint.
- Reiter's syndrome occurs in response to a gut infection or a venereal infection (see Puzzle 18).
- Rheumatic fever occurs after a streptococcal infection (see Puzzle 28).

Endocrine
- Acromegaly describes a pituitary tumour that secretes growth hormone. Joint pain and arthritis may occur in patients with this condition.

Haematological
- Haemarthrosis may result from a bleeding tendency, such as the haemophilias.
- Gout (see Puzzle 29) may occur when a large tumour load is being broken down – as may be the case in the treatment of leukaemias.
- Sickle cell crisis can present with severe joint pain (see Puzzle 13).

Immune/idiopathic
Some have obvious infective or inflammatory triggers:
- enteropathic arthritis (occurring in association with Crohn's disease or ulcerative colitis) (see Puzzle 16)
- Reiter's syndrome (see Puzzle 18)
- rheumatic fever (see Puzzle 28)

Others do not:
- ankylosing spondylitis (see Puzzle 15)
- rheumatoid arthritis (RA) (see Puzzles 7 and 8)
- scleroderma
- SLE (see Puzzle 19)

Metabolic
- Gout occurs when there is excess urate production or reduced excretion. Crystals are deposited in the joints, as well as in other tissues.

Iatrogenic
- A variety of drugs can trigger gout (especially chemotherapeutic agents, which cause tissue breakdown).
- There is also a long list of drugs that can cause lupus-like syndromes.
- And remember – many drug reactions cause joint aches (arthralgia).

Neoplastic
- Breakdown of a large tumour burden can cause gout due to excess urate production (crystal arthropathy).
- Rarely, 'paraneoplastic' arthritis occurs. This describes arthritis in patients with cancer that is not explained on the basis of malignant infiltration.
- Tumour of joints (eg, chondrosarcomas) can cause joint pain and swelling.

Remember
- Rheumatology isn't just about the joints.
- All diseases with an auto-immune component tend to be associated with blood vessel inflammation (vasculitis) and thus all organs can be affected.
- Many conditions are also systemic – eg, infections, gout (affects diverse organs).

PUZZLE 2   OSTEOARTHRITIS

This puzzle is a crossword. The solutions are all features of osteoarthritis (OA) except for one, which is a feature of another arthritis. What is this condition?

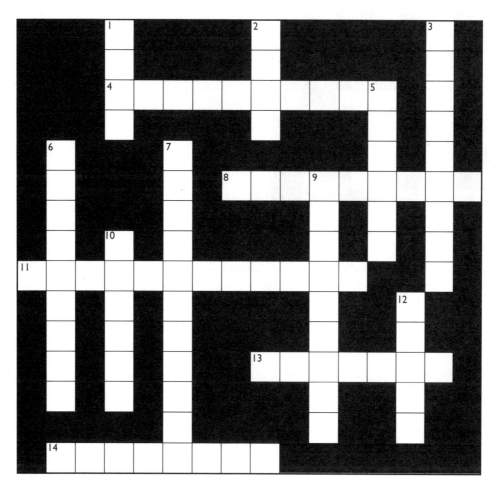

Down

1. Joint commonly affected in obese women (housemaid's _ _ _ is bursitis above this) (4)
2. and **6 Down**. Subchondral X-ray changes include formation of small cavities, each being a _ _ _ and increased 'whiteness' recognised as _ _ _ (4,9)
3. Bony nodules over the distal interphalangeal (DIP) joints (9)
5. Radial subluxation may give this shape to the hand (6)
6. See **2 Down**
7. Calcified cartilaginous growths at the margin of affected joints (11)
9. OA is characterised by loss of articular _ _ _ (9)
10. Joint stiffness typically lasts no longer than _ _ _ minutes (6)
12. May be illustrated by loss of _ _ _ space on X-ray (5)

Across

4. Inflammation at ligamentous bone junction (10)
8. Similar to **5 Down**, but found at the proximal interphalangeal (PIP) joints (9)
11. Surgical procedure to improve joint function (12)
13. Medication may cause lethargy secondary to _ _ _ (7)
14. A bulge test at the knee may reveal this (8)

PUZZLE 2 OSTEOARTHRITIS

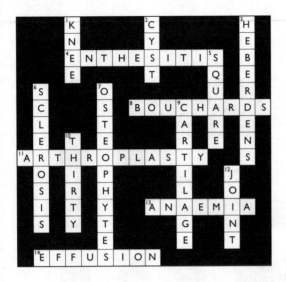

The odd one out is **enthesitis** (4 Across). This is seen in ankylosing spondylitis (AS). What are the other features of AS? See Puzzle 15.

Clinical features

- Osteoarthritis (OA) is characterised by loss of articular cartilage with accompanying periarticular bone responses.
- It is the most common form of arthritis, affecting about 50% of those over 60 years of age.
- It has a multifactorial aetiology, and may be the result of a primary abnormality or be secondary to a predisposing factor such as trauma ('wear and tear') or bone disease.
- Pathogenesis may be summarised as follows:

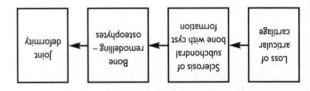

- Secondary inflammation occurs, and may be exacerbated by the release of small cartilage fragments into the joint space.
- Effusions may also result.
- OA results in stiff, painful joints with limited movement.
- The small joints of the hands, knees and hips are commonly involved in an asymmetrical pattern.
- There are no systemic features.
- Movement worsens pain, but paradoxically relieves stiffness.

Diagnosis

- Diagnosis is made clinically, although X-rays may reveal characteristic features such as joint space narrowing, osteophytes, subchondral sclerosis and cyst formation.

Treatment

- Treatment focuses around physical measures, (eg, weight loss, and physiotherapy to aid mobility) and medical measures (eg, NSAIDs to dampen inflammation and analgesic drugs such as paracetamol).
- There may be a role for glucosamine (mechanism of action is unclear).
- Surgery may be needed (eg, osteotomy, arthrodesis, arthroplasty or joint replacement).

PUZZLE 2 OSTEOARTHRITIS

PUZZLE 3   SPONDYLOSIS

What is spondylosis?

Unravel the anagram to find out:

HOT-TO-TROT FISH INSPIRE EASE (14,2,3,5)

Spondylosis is:

OSTEOARTHRITIS OF THE SPINE

PUZZLE 3 SPONDYLOSIS

Spondylosis is another name for osteoarthritis (OA) of the intervertebral discs.

- There are four joints in the spine: the main two are the intervertebral (disc) and synovial facet joints; the others are the atlanto-axial and sacroiliac joints.
- Spinal OA is like any other OA – there is cartilage loss and increased bone turnover. Loss of disc space causes foraminal encroachment and thus nerve compression, which is made worse by the presence of osteophytes (which also restrict movement). Disc rupture/prolapse may cause similar effects.
- OA of the spine can also cause spinal cord compression through disc rupture and osteophytic narrowing of the central canal (causing spinal stenosis).

PUZZLE 4   SEROPOSITIVE AND SERONEGATIVE ARTHRITIDES

Some rheumatological diseases have readily detectable auto-antibodies, and are known as the seropositive arthritides. Others don't, and thus are known as the seronegative arthritides.

Can you attract the right diseases to the positive and negative poles of the magnet? One is not commonly associated with joint disease… Which is it?

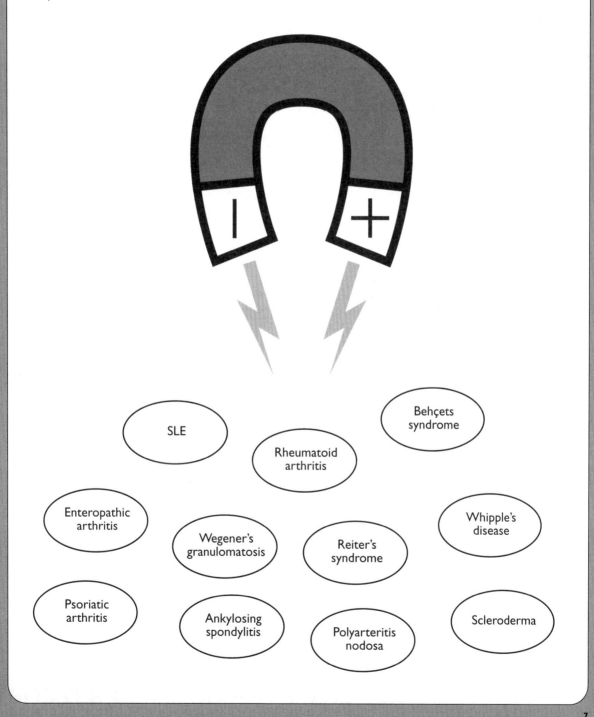

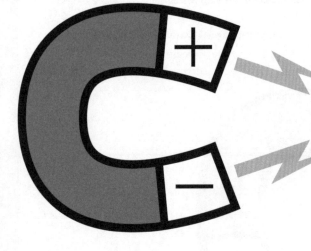

Seropositive arthritides

RA • SLE • Scleroderma • Wegener's granulomatosis

Seronegative arthritides

Ankylosing spondylitis • Behçets syndrome • Enteropathic arthritis • Polyarteritis nodosa (PAN) • Psoriatic arthritis • Reiter's syndrome • Whipple's disease

The disease not commonly associated with joint disease is Wegener's granulomatosis.

Seropositive arthritides

- RA – rheumatoid factor is an IgM antibody (rarely IgG). The former is detected with the sheep red-cell agglutination test (SCAT, Rose–Waaler test) or the latex agglutination/differential agglutination test (DAT).
- SLE – the presence of anti-dsDNA antibodies is highly specific for SLE. Anti-DNA histone antibodies cause 'LE cells' to appear; these particularly increase in drug-induced SLE. Anti-smooth muscle cell antibodies are also very specific, but (unlike anti-dsDNA) their titre doesn't change with disease activity. See Puzzle 19.
- Scleroderma/systemic sclerosis (SSc) – a variety of auto-antibodies may be found in this disorder. Extractable nuclear antigens (ENAs) are raised in this and in 'mixed connective tissue disease' – a crossover between diseases like SLE and SSc. See Puzzle 21.
- Wegener's granulomatosis – an auto-immune disease that is ANCA (anti-neutrophil cytoplasmic antibodies) positive. Joint pain is not a major feature in general.

Seronegative arthritides

- Ankylosing spondylitis – see Puzzle 15.
- Behçet's syndrome – this condition is of unknown origin and results in recurrent arthritis and mouth and genital ulceration. In addition, there may be encephalitis, myocarditis and thrombophlebitis.
- Enteropathic arthritis – see Puzzle 16.
- Polyarteritis nodosa (PAN) – note that hepatitis B surface antigen is sometimes found. See Puzzle 26.
- Psoriatic arthritis – see Puzzle 17.
- Reiter's syndrome – see Puzzle 18.
- Whipple's disease – this is a cause of malabsorption that usually occurs in men. The condition is associated with arthritis, cachexia and lymphadenopathy. A jejunal biopsy demonstrates PAS (periodic acid Schiff)-positive glycoprotein granules.

All of these are more common in men than in women. All lack clear auto-antibody patterns, and most are HLA-B27-associated. They tend to be asymmetrical. The other main differences are listed in the Puzzle 5.

PUZZLE 4 SEROPOSITIVE AND SERONEGATIVE ARTHRITIDES

PUZZLE 5 SEROPOSITIVE AND SERONEGATIVE FEATURES

Oops! This table has been wrongly filled in. Some lines are right, but other bits have gone wrong. Can you correct the table?

	Seronegative	Seropositive	Correct?
Symmetrical?	Yes	No	
Sacroiliacs commonly hit?	Yes	No	
Spine effect?	Ankylosis	Subluxation	
Eyes?	Scleritis/episcleritis/ keratoconjunctivitis sicca	Anterior uveitis/ conjunctivitis	
HLA-B27?	Often	Not associated	
Heart affected?	Pericarditis	Aortic regurgitation	
Skin associations?	Psoriasis, keratoderma, mucosal ulceration	Cutaneous nodules	
Vasculitis?	Yes	No	
GI association?	Yes – mucosal ulceration can lead to inflammatory bowel disease	No	
Gastric ulcer involvement?	Rare	Common	

	Seronegative	Seropositive
Symmetrical?	No	Yes
Sacroiliacs commonly hit?	Yes	No
Spine effect?	Ankylosis	Subluxation
Eyes?	Anterior uveitis/ conjunctivitis	Scleritis/episcleritis/ keratoconjunctivitis sicca
HLA-B27?	Often	Not associated
Heart affected?	Aortic regurgitation	Pericarditis
Skin associations?	Psoriasis, keratoderma, mucosal ulceration	Cutaneous nodules
Vasculitis?	No	Yes
GI association?	Yes – mucosal ulceration can lead to inflammatory bowel disease	No
Gastric ulcer involvement?	Common	Rare

_____

_____   _____

_____   _____

_____   _____

_____   _____

_____   _____

_____   _____

_____   _____

PUZZLE 6 ASSOCIATED FEATURES OF RHEUMATOLOGICAL DISEASES

Many rheumatological diseases have associated features. It is important to ask about these since they can provide important clues to the diagnosis. You seek the following. Can you link them to the signs and possible diagnoses?

	Signs	Diagnosis
1. Skin changes	Subcutaneous nodules	SLE
	Butterfly rash	Scleroderma
	Tight skin	RA
2. Changes in nails	Pitting	Fear of exams
	Nailfold infarcts	RA
	Bitten nails	Psoriatic arthropathy
3. Altered bowel habit	Yes	Rheumatic fever
		PAN
	No	Reiter's syndrome
		Ulcerative colitis
		RA
4. Urethral discharge	Yes	Septic arthritis
	No	Reiter's syndrome
	± Yes	RA
		Rheumatic fever

PUZZLE 6 ASSOCIATED FEATURES OF RHEUMATOLOGICAL DISEASES

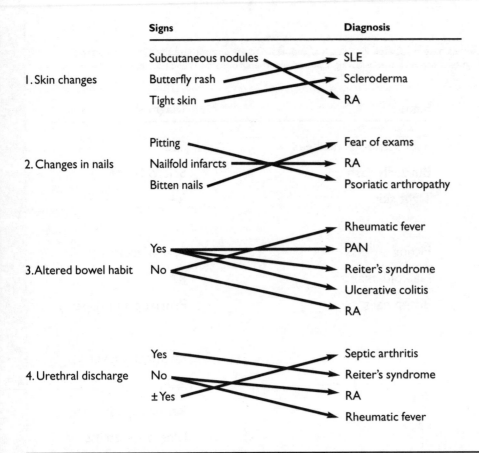

Signs		Diagnosis
1. Skin changes	Subcutaneous nodules	SLE
	Butterfly rash	Scleroderma
	Tight skin	RA
2. Changes in nails	Pitting	Fear of exams
	Nailfold infarcts	RA
	Bitten nails	Psoriatic arthropathy
3. Altered bowel habit	Yes	Rheumatic fever
	No	PAN
		Reiter's syndrome
		Ulcerative colitis
		RA
4. Urethral discharge	Yes	Septic arthritis
	No	Reiter's syndrome
	± Yes	RA
		Rheumatic fever

Skin changes

Subcutaneous nodules suggest RA, a butterfly rash occurs in SLE, psoriasis in psoriatic arthropathy, tight skin in scleroderma.

Nails

Nail pitting occurs in psoriasis, nailfold infarcts are seen with RA.

Altered bowel habit

Changes in bowel habit may suggest seronegative arthropathy related to inflammatory bowel disease, or small-bowel overgrowth with malabsorption in systemic sclerosis.

Urethral discharge

Think of Reiter's syndrome (see Puzzle 18).

Fever/recent weight loss

These are constitutional symptoms that may be especially associated with vasculitic diseases – especially RA, SLE, myositis and polyarteritis nodosa.

Eye pain or irritation

Keratoconjunctivitis sicca is associated with Sjögren's syndrome (see Puzzle 23). Think also of uveitis, which may complicate RA, ankylosing spondylitis and reactive arthritis.

Unusual sensations or loss of sensation in your limbs?

Neuropathies may complicate vasculitides.

PUZZLE 7   RHEUMATOID ARTHRITIS –
SYMPTOMS AND SIGNS

Here's a wordsearch about RA. Words may be read upwards, downwards, or diagonally in any direction. There are 10 features of RA: eight are articular and two are extra-articular. What are they?

For a bonus: three words link to form a three letter abbreviation meaning constipation. Also included is someone who would never get joint pain! Can you find them?

J	O	I	N	T	P	A	I	N	R	Z	F	B	H	O	B	E	N
M	E	L	T	O	V	F	E	E	A	S	C	A	D	I	B	N	O
U	O	E	Y	K	I	L	R	L	E	E	F	S	S	Y	O	K	I
L	U	R	B	M	N	K	G	U	T	R	T	I	H	I	U	R	T
N	S	I	N	F	P	B	U	I	L	R	J	T	S	D	T	O	A
A	C	J	H	I	U	H	I	O	A	E	A	U	R	S	O	L	X
R	L	I	L	E	N	N	A	L	P	P	F	E	U	N	N	A	U
D	E	E	N	O	T	G	K	D	O	F	U	F	I	R	N	S	L
E	W	R	N	R	V	I	S	N	E	I	F	O	D	V	I	E	B
V	A	M	E	R	C	T	E	T	L	N	O	P	S	C	E	H	U
I	S	L	I	M	R	D	N	I	I	D	O	C	X	A	R	T	S
A	R	R	E	E	A	I	U	N	E	F	D	P	O	S	E	G	T
T	I	E	Y	H	O	A	I	N	T	E	F	F	A	S	S	R	N
I	N	I	V	J	J	A	R	I	O	S	D	N	A	T	I	O	I
O	G	M	J	E	N	J	U	N	M	V	B	C	E	C	H	B	O
N	Y	Z	D	E	F	O	R	M	I	T	Y	R	F	S	S	Y	J
L	P	A	S	S	M	A	D	S	P	E	U	I	B	E	S	C	J
M	R	C	P	M	J	G	N	I	K	C	E	N	N	A	W	S	I

PUZZLE 7 RHEUMATOID ARTHRITIS – SYMPTOMS AND SIGNS

```
J O I N T P A I N . . . . . N
M L . . . . . . . . . B N O
U O Y . . . . . . . . O I
L R M . . . . . . I U T
N N P . . . . S T A
A I H . . U . O X
R N A . F . N U
D G D F . N L
E S E . I B
V T N . E U
I N I O R S
A R I F P E G T
T E O F A S R N
I V J N T O I
O E E H B O
N Z D E F O R M I T Y S Y J
S C
G N I K C E N N A W S
```

Articular features:

Boutonniere's (deformity of the fingers) • Joint effusion • Joint pain • Joint subluxation • Morning stiffness • Swan necking • Ulnar deviation • Z-deformity

Extra-articular features:

Fever • Lymphadenopathy

The three-letter abbreviation for constipation is:

BNO (bowels not open)

Someone who would never get joint pain is a:

CYBORG

RA is a chronic auto-immune disorder of unknown aetiology. It has a prevalence of 1–3% in the UK population, peaking between 30 and 55 years of age. It is more common in women (premenopausal women to men: 2:1) and there is an association with HLA-DR4.

- Synovial tissue is the main focus of inflammation in RA.
- RA is characterised by symmetrical polyarthritis, usually of the hands, elbows, shoulders, knees and feet.
- Characteristic radiological findings include: soft tissue swelling; joint space narrowing; periarticular osteoporosis; cysts; and, rarely, atlanto-axial subluxation.
- 70% of patients have extra-articular involvement of the eyes, blood, lungs, heart and many other organs.
- The diagnosis is usually clinical, but investigations may reveal a normochromic/normocytic anaemia and thrombocytosis.
- Rheumatoid factor (RF) is positive in 70% of cases and anti-nuclear antibodies (ANA) in 30%.

Articular features

- Boutonniere's deformity of the fingers (flexion deformity of the proximal interphalangeal joint with extension contractures of both metacarpophalangeal and terminal interphalangeal joints); = 'button workers' finger'.
- Joint effusion
- Joint pain
- Joint subluxation
- Morning stiffness
- Swan necking (hyperextension of the proximal interphalangeal joint with fixed flexion of both the metacarpophalangeal and terminal interphalangeal joints)
- Ulnar deviation
- Z-deformity of the thumb (flexion of the terminal interphalangeal joint and extension of the proximal interphalangeal joint)

Symptoms related to joints

- Carpal tunnel syndrome (see Puzzle 33)
- Atlanto-axial subluxation (if this joint becomes unstable, the odontoid peg can flap free and extension of the neck can make it press on the brainstem. This can be lethal! Be careful, therefore, in preparing those with RA for a general anaesthetic: you may need imaging first, and cervical protection. Otherwise, RA + GA may = RIP!)

Extra-articular features

- General systemic features
  – fever
  – malaise
  – fatigue
- Sjogren's syndrome (see Puzzle 23)
- Nodule-related. Nodules can occur anywhere causing organ disease, especially:
  – skin nodules (painless subcutaneous: extensor forearm surface)
  – rheumatoid lung
  – myocardial disease
- Eye
  – episcleritis
  – scleritis
  – uveitis
- Haematological
  – anaemia (caused by chronic disease, NSAID-induced gastrointestinal blood loss or Coomb's-positive haemolytic anaemia)
  – Felty's syndrome (RA, splenomegaly and neutropenia)
  – thrombocytosis
- Serositis
  – pleural effusion
  – pericarditis

PUZZLE 7 RHEUMATOID ARTHRITIS – SYMPTOMS AND SIGNS

PUZZLE 8 RHEUMATOID ARTHRITIS – MANAGEMENT

A multidisciplinary approach is essential for the efficient and effective treatment of RA. Treatment is guided by the following simple injunction: STOP THE SYNOVITIS. A variety of drug classes can be used to this end.

The table below has become muddled. Can you draw up a correct version using the blank template? Match each drug to its mechanism of action, one major side effect and how patients should be monitored.

Drug	Mechanism of action	Side-effect	Monitoring
NSAIDs	Prevent signal transduction post T-cell activation	↓ Bone marrow	Full ophthalmic examination before treatment and then every 3–6 months
Sulfasalazine	Unknown	Liver cirrhosis	FBC monthly
Methotrexate	Purine anti-metabolite	Retinopathy	FBC and LFTs monthly for 6 months, then at 3-monthly intervals
Cyclosporin	Dissociates immune complexes and inhibits T-cell activation	Peptic ulceration	None
Gold	Folate antagonist	Proteinuria	FBC and urine every 1–2 weeks for first 5 months, then monthly
Azathioprine	Inhibits receptor cycling and decreases cytokine production	Gingival hypertrophy	FBC and LFTs weekly for first month, then monthly
Penicillamine	Cyclooxygenase (COX) inhibitor	↓ Spermatogenesis	Test urine and FBC before each IM injection
Hydroxychloro-quine	Inhibits prostaglandin production	Thrombocytopenia	Renal function and LFTs every 2–3 weeks

Drug	Mechanism of action	Side-effect	Monitoring

Drug	Mechanism of action	Side-effect	Monitoring
NSAIDs	Cyclooxygenase (COX) inhibitor	Peptic ulceration	None
Sulfasalazine	Inhibits prostaglandin production	↓Spermatogenesis	FBC and LFTs monthly for 6 months, then at 3-monthly intervals
Methotrexate	Folate antagonist	Liver cirrhosis	FBC and LFTs weekly for first month, then monthly
Cyclosporin	Prevent signal transduction post T-cell activation	Gingival hypertrophy	Renal function and LFTs every 2–3 weeks
Gold	Unknown	Proteinuria	Test urine and FBC before each IM injection
Azathioprine	Purine anti-metabolite	↓Bone marrow	FBC monthly
Penicillamine	Dissociates immune complexes and inhibits T-cell activation	Thrombocytopenia	FBC and urine every 1–2 weeks for first 5 months, then monthly
Hydroxychloro-quine	Inhibits receptor cycling and decreases cytokine production	Retinopathy	Full ophthalmic examination before treatment and then every 3–6 months

1. Stop the synovitis

This is primarily achieved with anti-inflammatory drugs, disease-modifying anti-rheumatic drugs (DMARDs) and corticosteroids.

Anti-inflammatory drugs are effective at providing symptomatic relief, but do not affect disease progression. However, if given early in the disease process, DMARDs are able to prevent some of the irreversible effects of long-term joint inflammation.

Corticosteroids are also effective at providing symptomatic relief, but their role in management is controversial because of their many side-effects.

2. Prevent deformity

This is the second goal of treatment

Inflamed joints should be rested, but should also be put through a passive range of movements each day to prevent joint deformity and increase function.

Replacement or reconstruction of joints is indicated if pain and loss of function have failed to respond to drug therapy and physiotherapy.

Prognosis of RA

This is variable. After 10 years, 10% of patients will be severely crippled and 25% will go into remission. The other patients will lie somewhere between these two extremes.

Interestingly, the long-term prognosis tends to be better when the onset is sudden.

PUZZLE 9   RHEUMATIC SYMPTOMS – I. PAIN

Three important symptoms in rheumatological disease are joint pain, stiffness and swelling. Joint pain may arise because of articular and/or extra-articular factors. Can you connect the factors causing joint pain with their appropriate class?

Erosion/loss of joint cartilage

Soft-tissue injury

Articular causes   Change in composition of the synovial fluid

Bursitis

Infection

Tendonitis

Referred pain

Extra-articular causes   Enthesitis

Synovitis

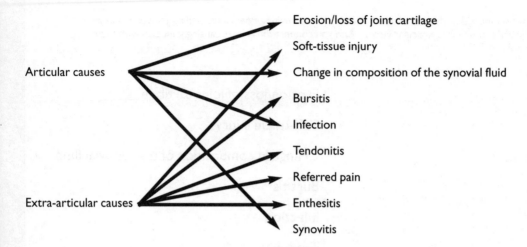

Articular causes

Extra-articular causes

Erosion/loss of joint cartilage
Soft-tissue injury
Change in composition of the synovial fluid
Bursitis
Infection
Tendonitis
Referred pain
Enthesitis
Synovitis

Infected joints are a MEDICAL EMERGENCY! Call for senior help!

Key questions about the joint pain

1. Where is it?
2. How long does it last?
3. Is it persistent/intermittent?
4. What is its character?
5. Where does it radiate?
6. Relieving and exacerbating factors
7. How does it affect your mobility?

PUZZLE 10 RHEUMATIC SYMPTOMS –
II. JOINT STIFFNESS

Causes of joint stiffness can be divided into two categories: mechanical or inflammatory. Each category differs in its presentation.

Which of the following statements best describes a mechanical cause for joint stiffness and which best describes an inflammatory cause?

Statement 1.

Joint stiffness is worse in the morning and usually gets better throughout the day, although it can be exacerbated by movement.

Statement 2.

Joint stiffness usually lasts no longer than 30 minutes in the morning, tends to get worse towards the end of the day and improves with movement.

PUZZLE 10 RHEUMATIC SYMPTOMS – II. JOINT STIFFNESS

Inflammatory cause

Statement 1. Joint stiffness of an inflammatory cause is usually worse in the morning and gets better throughout the day, although it can be exacerbated by movement. Causative diseases include RA, seronegative arthropathies and polymyalgia rheumatica (PMR).

Mechanical cause

Statement 2. Joint stiffness of a mechanical cause usually lasts no longer than 30 minutes in the morning, tends to get worse towards the end of the day and improves with movement. Causative diseases/factors include OA and trauma.

Key questions about joint stiffness

1. When does it occur?
2. How long does it last?
3. How severe is it?

PUZZLE 10 RHEUMATIC SYMPTOMS – II. JOINT STIFFNESS

PUZZLE 11 RHEUMATIC SYMPTOMS – III. JOINT SWELLING

Doctor Smith has eight patients. Using the following table of clinical features, can you help him discover their diagnoses?

- Bob, Nick and Jed have all suffered from infections.
- Mildred, Alex and Jed have all suffered rapid joint swelling.
- Lucy has suffered both chronic and intermittent joint swellings.
- Neither Mildred nor Jed remember hurting themselves.
- Both Bob and Nick have suffered diarrhoea, but Nick also has red eyes.
- Dave has a stiff back and HLA-B27/DR3.
- All have 'seronegative arthropathies', except for one woman.
- Jed does not have crystals in his joints.
- Simon has scaly leisons over his extensor surfaces.

The patterns of presentation of joint swelling are as follows:

Disease	Acute swelling	Progressive swelling	Intermittent swelling	Chronic swelling
Enteropathic arthritis			✓	
RA			✓	✓
Reiter's syndrome		✓	✓	
Gout	✓			
Septic arthritis	✓			
Psoriatic arthritis			✓	
Ankylosing spondylitis				✓
Trauma	✓			

PUZZLE 11 RHEUMATIC SYMPTOMS – III. JOINT SWELLING

Patient	Diagnosis
Bob	Enteropathic arthritis
Lucy	RA
Nick	Reiter's syndrome
Mildred	Gout
Jed	Septic arthritis
Simon	Psoriatic arthritis
Dave	Ankylosing spondylitis
Alex	Trauma

The following are all causes of joint swelling:

- enteropathic arthritis (see Puzzle 16)
- RA (see Puzzles 7 and 8)
- Reiter's syndrome (see Puzzle 18)
- gout (see Puzzle 29)
- septic arthritis (see Puzzle 27)
- psoriatic arthritis (see Puzzle 17)
- ankylosing spondylitis (see Puzzle 15)
- trauma (can affect any joint)

Key questions about joint swelling

1. Is it acute or chronic?
2. Is it intermittent or progressive?

PUZZLE 11 RHEUMATIC SYMPTOMS – III. JOINT SWELLING

PUZZLE 12 CHRONIC JUVENILE ARTHRITIS – PAUCIARTICULAR ARTHRITIS

Chronic juvenile arthritis (CJA) is a group of conditions that present in childhood with arthritis lasting for at least 6 months. The major subtypes include pauciarticular arthritis, polyarticular arthritis and Still's disease. CJA is a clinical diagnosis and management aims to maintain joint mobility and avoid or control complications.

The passage below is about pauciarticular arthritis. Fill in the missing words (shown below).

Pauciarticular arthritis accounts for about _ _ _ of all cases of CJA and commonly affects _ _ _ under the age of _ _ _ years. Patients typically present with _ _ _, mild _ _ _ that most commonly affects the _ _ _, followed by the _ _ _, wrist and elbows. Up to _ _ _ joints can be affected. Systemic symptoms are usually _ _ _. Seventy percent of patients, who are usually _ _ _, are ANA- _ _ _. The remaining 30%, who are usually _ _ _, are often HLA-B27- _ _ _. The disease carries a _ _ _ risk of developing chronic _ _ _ and regular examination with a _ _ _ is required to screen for this. The prognosis is _ _ _ as the arthritis usually resolves _ _ _.

Missing from the text are:

50% • ankle • arthritis • asymmetrical • boys • completely • excellent • five • four • girls • girls • high • iridocyclitis • knee • minimal • positive • positive • slit-lamp

PUZZLE 12 CHRONIC JUVENILE ARTHRITIS – PAUCIARTICULAR ARTHRITIS

The completed passage:

Pauciarticular arthritis accounts for about **50%** of all cases of CJA and commonly affects **girls** under the age of **five** years. Patients typically present with **asymmetrical**, mild **arthritis** that most commonly affects the **knee**, followed by the **ankle**, wrist and elbows. Up to **four** joints can be affected. Systemic symptoms are usually **minimal**. 70% of patients, who are usually **girls**, are ANA-**positive**. The remaining 30%, who are usually **boys**, are often HLA-B27-**positive**. The disease carries a **high** risk of developing chronic **iridocyclitis** and regular examination with a **slit-lamp** is required to screen for this. The prognosis **is excellent** as the arthritis usually resolves **completely**.

Definition

Pauciarticular arthritis implies the involvement of up to four joints. It is the most common type of CJA.

Clinical features

- More common in girls than boys (70%:30%).
- Usually occurs between ages 2 and 3 years, rare after 10 years of age.
- Characteristically affects the large joints (knees, ankles, wrists, elbows), but virtually never begins in the hips.
- Usually asymmetrical.
- Associated with uveitis (high risk of iridocyclitis).
- Systemic manifestations (other than uveitis) are characteristically absent.

Diagnosis

Clinically, patients must have four or fewer joints involved. Anti-nuclear antibodies (ANAs) are frequently present, but other antibodies are absent. X-rays may be useful.

Prognosis

Pauciarticular arthritis resolves in 6 months, but 20% of cases recur. Uveitis may be a problem.

Treatment

- NSAIDs
- Steroid injection
- Physiotherapy
- Ophthalmology review for uveitis. This is a potentially serious complication.

PUZZLE 12 CHRONIC JUVENILE ARTHRITIS – PAUCIARTICULAR ARTHRITIS

PUZZLE 13 CHRONIC JUVENILE ARTHRITIS – POLYARTICULAR ARTHRITIS

In this puzzle the answers to the questions are true or false. If the answer is true, take the letter from the true column; if the answer is false, take the letter from the false column. At the end you will have 10 letters. Rearrange these letters to give another cause of bone pain in children.

		True	False
1.	In polyarticular arthritis, systemic steroids should be given early in the disease	F	L
2.	In polyarticular juvenile arthritis, fewer than four joints are usually affected	G	E
3.	Uveitis is less common in polyarticular disease than in pauciarticular arthritis	L	A
4.	Internal organ involvement is common in polyarticular juvenile arthritis	P	C
5.	Polyarticular juvenile arthritis is more common in females than in males	S	R
6.	In polyarticular juvenile arthritis, the joints are usually affected asymmetrically	A	L
7.	Polyarticular juvenile arthritis usually starts within the first year of life	R	I
8.	NSAIDs are useful in treating polyarticular juvenile arthritis	E	P
9.	Patients with polyarticular juvenile arthritis do not usually present with high fever	C	O
10.	In polyarticular juvenile arthritis, patients with severe arthritis have a good prognosis	R	K

1. False (L)

2. False (E)

3. True (L)

4. False (C)

5. True (S)

6. False (L)

7. False (I)

8. True (E)

9. True (C)

10. False (K)

The hidden cause of bone pain is SICKLE CELL (anaemia). Patients with sickle cell anaemia may have joint and bone pain caused by vaso-occlusive crises. Many patients also suffer from the long-term consequences of this, with avascular necrosis of the femoral heads or collapsed vertebral bodies. Patients with sickle cell anaemia are also more prone to osteomyelitis due to *Salmonella* infection.

Definition

More than four affected joints during the first 6 months of illness.

Clinical features

- More frequent in females than in males.
- Bimodal age distribution: the first peak in incidence is between the ages of 2 and 5 years, and the second peak is between 10 and 14 years.
- Usually starts with two joints and then spreads to involve five or more joints before the end of 6 months. Joint involvement is usually symmetrical, with the knees, wrists, and ankles most frequently affected.
- Uveitis can occur, although it is much less common than in children with pauciarticular CJA.
- Internal organ involvement is rare.

Diagnosis

Clinically, more than four joints must be affected during the first 6 months of disease. There are no characteristic laboratory findings, although patients may have positive auto-antibodies.

Prognosis

Young children with progressive polyarthritis are at risk for lifelong disability.

Treatment

- NSAIDs are a useful primary treatment.
- If no response, patients may need sulfasalazine.
- Consider intra-articular steroids.

PUZZLE 13 CHRONIC JUVENILE ARTHRITIS – POLYARTICULAR ARTHRITIS

PUZZLE 14 CHRONIC JUVENILE ARTHRITIS –
STILL'S DISEASE

When combined with the mystery letter in the centre, the letters in each section of the circle will form six features that may be seen on first presentation of Still's disease. Can you find the features of Still's disease and identify the mystery letter? What other important presenting symptom have we missed out?

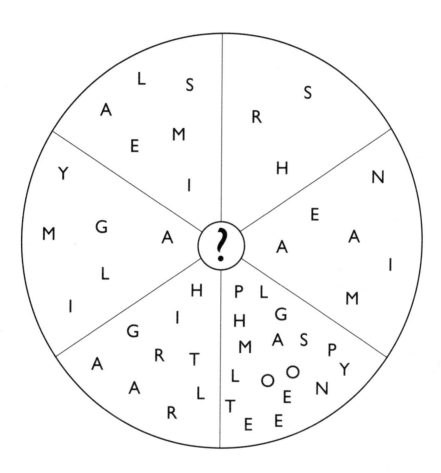

PUZZLE 14 CHRONIC JUVENILE ARTHRITIS – STILL'S DISEASE

Another important systemic symptom is daily spiking fever.

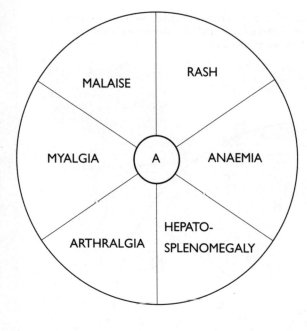

Still's disease is a systemic-onset, juvenile RA. Patients have intermittent fever, rash, arthritis and organ involvement.

Clinical features

- Affects both sexes equally.
- Cases are distributed throughout childhood.
- Arthralgias are common. Disease in the wrists, knees and ankles is most typical. Unlike the pauciarticular and polyarticular subtypes of CJA, the arthritis of Still's disease can begin in the hips.
- Micrognathia and cervical spine fusion are commonly present in children who have chronic systemic symptoms.
- Patients may have multiple extra-articular manifestations. These include fevers, a salmon-pink rash, hepatomegaly, splenomegaly and lymphadenopathy. Furthermore, patients can have pericardial and pleural effusions and other cardiac problems.

Diagnosis

Clinically, patients have the combination of intermittent daily fevers higher than 38.5°C and arthritis. FBC shows anaemia, increased WCC and increased platelets. ESR and CRP are elevated. Auto-antibodies are rare.

Course and prognosis

Patients may have persistent problems. Prognosis is worse than in the other types of CJA.

Treatment

- NSAIDs alone are effective for many children with systemic-onset CJA.
- Consider second-line drugs such as DMARDS (disease-modifying anti-rheumatic drugs) if symptoms do not resolve, or corticosteroids to control severe symptoms.

28

PUZZLE 15 ANKYLOSING SPONDYLITIS

This puzzle is a tricky sort of crossword about ankylosing spondylitis (AS). To make life difficult, you aren't told which answers go where.

The solutions are all features/treatments of ankylosing spondylitis except one, which is a feature of another seronegative arthropathy. What is this condition?

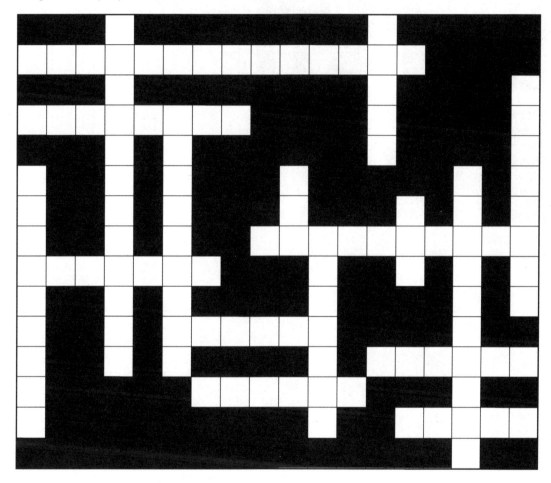

Clues

1. This age group of men is usually affected (5)

2. It mainly involves the -_ _ _ skeleton and large proximal joints (5)

3. Patients suffer from morning _ _ _ (9)

4. Spine X-ray may remind you of this exotic grass (6)

5,6. Radiographs may show _ _ _ and _ _ _ of the margins of the sacroiliac joints (7,9)

7. Inflammation at a ligamentous bone junction (10)

8,9. On inspection of the spine, there is loss of the lumbar _ _ _ and increased outward bend or _ _ _ (8,8)

10. Fixed _ _ _ of the hips may result (7)

11. Compensatory _ _ _ of the neck may lead to a 'shepherd's crook' shape to the spine (14)

12. This cause of painful micturition may be associated (10)

13. 25% have this eye involvement (6)

14,15. Raised as a blood test marker of inflammation. Two common tests (3,3)

16. _ _ _ are particularly effective in reducing night pain and morning stiffness (6)

17. Folate antagonist that may help peripheral arthritis (12)

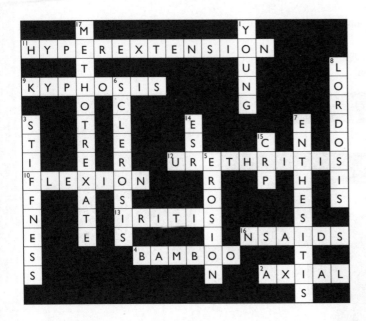

The odd one out is:

Urethritis (clue 13), which is a feature of Reiter's syndrome. What are the other characteristic features of Reiter's syndrome? See Puzzle 18.

Ankylosing spondylitis is a chronic inflammatory disease of unknown aetiology, affecting 0.5–1% of the population. It is more common among young Caucasian men and is associated with HLA-B27, as are most of the seronegative arthropathies.

It mainly affects the axial skeleton causing lower back pain, but also causes peripheral arthritis of large proximal joints (such as the shoulders) and enthesitis (inflammation at the site where ligaments, tendons and the joint capsule attach to bone).

Spine stiffening leads to a hunchback appearance, with hyperextension (so that the person can still look up) causing a 'shepherd's crook' spine shape. Restriction in spine movement can be debilitating and can limit chest expansion (and is thus a cause of respiratory failure).

Extra-articular manifestations include fever, anaemia, acute anterior uveitis, aortic valve incompetence, bilateral upper lobe fibrosis and secondary amyloidosis.

Diagnosis

The diagnosis is primarily clinical, although characteristic radiographic changes may be seen as the disease progresses. These include:

- squaring, bony bridging and fusion of adjacent vertebrae giving the spine a 'bamboo' appearance
- erosion and sclerosis at vertebral bony margins (Romanus sign)
- enthesitis and secondary ossification leading to proliferate bone margins, spicules and spurs at ligamentous bony junctions (commonly the pelvis, plantar fascia and Achilles tendons)

Treatment

The aims of management are to minimize spinal deformities and maximize skeletal mobility. Patients should be encouraged to keep mobile. Drugs do not halt the disease process, but NSAIDs may reduce pain and stiffness. About 10% of patients develop progressive crippling disease. Most patients, however, lead a normal life and have a normal life expectancy.

PUZZLE 16 ENTEROPATHIC ARTHRITIS

This is a shape puzzle. Enteropathic arthritis is a seronegative (HLA-B27-associated) arthritis. Fit this jigsaw together to identify three causes and two joints that are often involved in this disease. What other joint is commonly involved?

Clue: The pieces join together to form a pyramid.

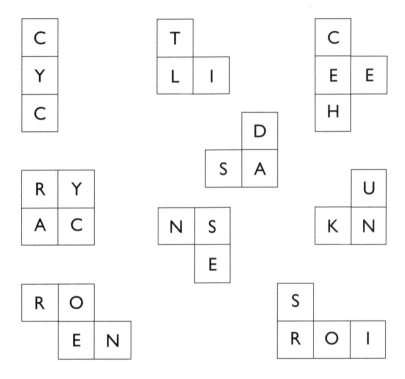

PUZZLE 16 ENTEROPATHIC ARTHRITIS

In the puzzle are:

Crohn's • UC • Dysentery • Knee • Sacroiliac

The other commonly involved joint is the ankle.

```
            U  C
         K  N  E  E
      C  R  O  H  N  S
   D  Y  S  E  N  T  E  R  Y
S  A  C  R  O  I  L  I  A  C
```

Enteropathic arthritis is associated with gut disease. It can occur following an episode of dysentery (especially infections with *Shigella, Salmonella, Yersinia* and *Campylobacter*) or in association with inflammatory bowel disease (IBD: ulcerative colitis [UC] and Crohn's disease [approx 10–15% of patients are affected]). Management is thus focused on controlling these diseases.

- The arthritis usually affects large joints and is a mono- or asymmetrical oligoarthritis, usually affecting the knee or the ankle.
- The severity of joint involvement parallels the activity of the IBD.
- The prognosis is generally good for both IBD-associated and dysentery-associated enteropathic arthritis, with attacks resolving within a few weeks. However, ankylosing spondylitis occurs in 5% of patients with IBD-associated arthritis.

PUZZLE 17 PSORIATIC ARTHRITIS

This link-letter puzzle is about psoriatic arthritis. Put the following letter groups into the boxes to produce four features (clinical, treatment, etc.) of psoriatic arthritis. We have already put in the 'I' to start you off...

IN   RO   RT   TT   GAT   TIS   GOA   RM   OL

TE   DS   HRI   NE   ENT   SE   ~~I~~   NSA   VE

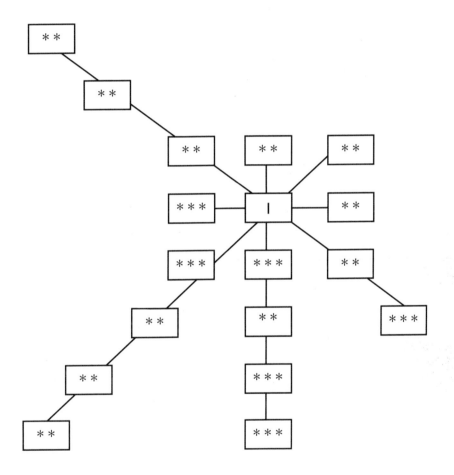

PUZZLE 17   PSORIATIC ARTHRITIS

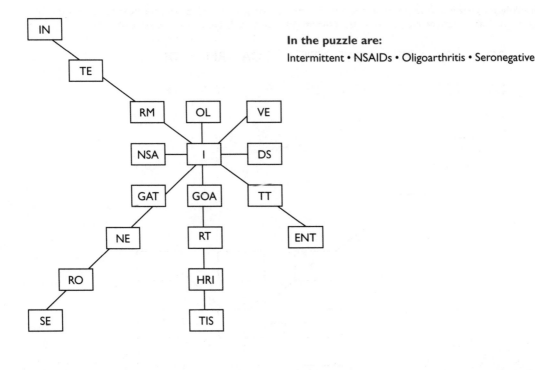

In the puzzle are:
Intermittent • NSAIDs • Oligoarthritis • Seronegative

PUZZLE 17   PSORIATIC ARTHRITIS

Psoriatic arthritis is a seronegative arthropathy (HLA-B27-associated) that affects approximately 5% of patients with psoriasis; those with nail disease are particularly susceptible. Males and females are equally affected, although the axial spine is more commonly affected in men and a symmetrical polyarthritis (like RA) occurs more frequently in women. The middle-aged (30–55 years) are the most common age group affected.

- There are several types that affect different groups of joints, ranging from the small joints of the hand to the sacroiliac joints. These types are an asymmetrical oligo- or mono-articular arthropathy, a type similar to RA in distribution and arthritis mutilans.
- Psoriatic arthritis is generally mild and intermittent, and spontaneous remission may occur.
- There does not appear to be any association between the extent of skin and nail involvement and the severity of the arthritis.
- Radiographs may reveal bony erosions and periarticular osteoporosis, particularly of the terminal interphalangeal joints.
- Ocular symptoms (eg, uveitis) are rarely associated.
- Management is symptomatic, with analgesia and NSAIDs.

PUZZLE 18   REACTIVE ARTHRITIS AND REITER'S SYNDROME

Reactive arthritis is the name given to arthritis of the large joints following enteric or venereal infections.

Unscramble the anagrams below to reveal four gastrointestinal infections and one venereal infection that can cause reactive arthritis:

1. SAGE HILL (8)

2. A SMALL NOEL (10)

3. IN ANY RISE (8)

4. COPYCAT RAMBLE (13)

5. MAYA CHILD (9)

Reiter's syndrome is reactive arthropathy plus two other clinical features. Unscramble the anagrams below to find the three main clinical features of Reiter's syndrome:

6. IRISH TART (9)

7. TRUE HIT SIR (10)

8. I CONVICT JUSTIN (14)

PUZZLE 18 REACTIVE ARTHRITIS AND REITER'S SYNDROME

The causes of reactive arthritis are:

1. SHIGELLA

2. SALMONELLA

3. YERSININA

4. CAMPYLOBACTER

5. CHLAMYDIA

The gut infection bacteria form some of the causes of enteropathic arthritis (see Puzzle 16).

The clinical features of Reiter's syndrome are:

6. ARTHRITIS

7. URETHRITIS

8. CONJUNCTIVITIS

Reactive arthritis is arthritis of the large joints following enteric or venereal infections. Reactive arthritis may also be associated with:

- iritis
- enthesopathy (plantar fasciitis, Achilles tendonitis)
- circinate balanitis (painless lesions on the glans penis)
- keratoderma blennorrhagica (scaling and papules on the palms, and soles that are indistinguishable from those seen in pustular psoriasis)

Reiter's syndrome is reactive arthropathy occurring with:

- urethritis (associated with dysuria and a sterile urethral discharge)
- conjunctivitis (occurs in one third of patients and is often mild with bilateral involvement)

The typical case is a young man who presents with an acute arthritis within 4 weeks of acquiring an enteric or venereal infection. The most common cause is genital infection with *Chlamydia trachomatis*. The joints of the lower limbs are typically affected in an asymmetrical pattern.

Management of reactive arthritis

Ensure that the predisposing infection has been adequately treated in both the patient and their partner.

Management is symptomatic, eg, NSAIDs and/or joint aspiration/intra-joint injection of corticosteroids for arthritis.

Prognosis of reactive arthritis/Reiter's syndrome

Most patients recover from the acute symptoms within a few months. However, 50% of patients develop recurrent arthritis, iritis or ankylosing spondylitis.

PUZZLE 18 REACTIVE ARTHRITIS AND REITER'S SYNDROME

PUZZLE 19   JOIN THE DOTS TO FIND
A SICK INSECT

What skin condition does the insect represent, and with what disease is it associated?

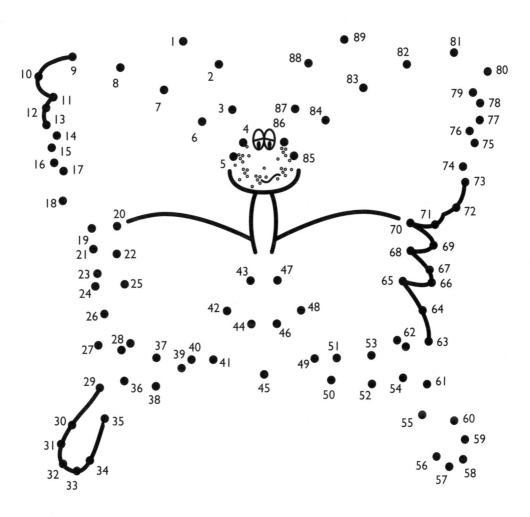

PUZZLE 19 JOIN THE DOTS TO FIND A SICK INSECT

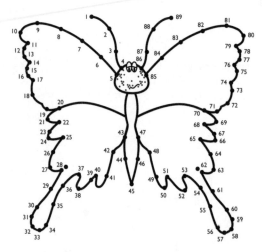

This is a 'butterfly rash' – found in SLE.

Epidemiology

SLE is mainly a disease of young women. It affects about 0.1% of the population, but is more common among Afro-Caribbeans.

The aetiology and pathogenesis are unknown, although it is postulated that immune complexes formed from auto-antibodies (eg, ANA, rheumatoid factor) cause cellular and tissue damage. The diagnosis is largely clinical and the disease tends to have a relapsing and remitting course.

Clinical features

SLE is associated with a vasculitis. Thus, pretty much any organ can be affected. Features are:

- constitutional
  – fever
  – malaise
- heart and circulation (40%)
  – pericarditis
  – endocarditis
  – valvular lesions (sterile 'mirantic' or Libman–Sacks endocarditis – often associated with anti-phospholipid antibodies [see Puzzle 20]
- dermatological (75%)
  – malar butterfly rash
  – mucosal ulcers
  – vasculitic rash
- central nervous system (60%)
  – psychosis
  – epilepsy
  – stroke
  – depression

- lungs (50%)
  – pleural effusion
  – restrictive lung defect
- rheumatological (90%)
  – arthralgia
  – symmetrical arthritis, often of the small joints
- blood (75%)
  – haemolytic anaemia
  – thrombocytopenia
- kidneys (50%)
  – nephritis

Diagnosis

- the patient needs to show a classical collection of clinical features
- blood tests, FBC and U&Es
- auto-antibodies, ANA, anti-dsDNA, anti-smooth muscle
- check complement levels (C3/C4)
- X-rays of affected joints
- consider renal biopsy if patient has renal impairment

Management

- NSAIDs – first-line in mild disease and for arthralgia
- hydroxychloroquine – second-line in mild disease and cutaneous involvement
- corticosteroids – mainstay of treatment for moderate/severe disease
- cyclophosphamide – helps renal disease
- topical steroids – used for discoid lupus

Prognosis

SLE is characterised by relapses and remissions. The 10-year survival is 90%. Infection followed by renal failure is the most common cause of death.

PUZZLE 20   ANTI-PHOSPHOLIPID SYNDROME

The following anagrams and questions are about anti-phospholipid syndrome (APS). Unscramble the anagrams to give three clinical features and two drugs that can be used to treat APS:

1. REST OK (6)

2. TRIBESMEN VIDEO SHOP (4,4,10)

3. RAIN BOOTS (9)

4. PAIN, SIR? (7)

5. RAF IN WAR (8)

PUZZLE 20 ANTI-PHOSPHOLIPID SYNDROME

1. STROKE

2. DEEP VEIN THROMBOSIS

3. ABORTIONS

4. ASPIRIN

5. WARFARIN

PUZZLE 20 ANTI-PHOSPHOLIPID SYNDROME

Pathology

APS may occur as a primary condition, or (more commonly) in association with SLE (or, rarely, other rheumatological conditions).

Two sorts of antibodies are found, which predispose to arterial and venous thrombosis:
– 'lupus anti-coagulant' helps to predict arterial thromboses
– auto-antibodies to β_2 glycoprotein 1 (anti-cardiolipin antibody [ACA], a phospholipid-binding protein)
The predictive value rises with titre.

Clinical features

Venous thrombosis
• Leg most commonly (and thus with pulmonary emboli)
• IVC/ileofemoral, axillary, retinal
• Budd–Chiari syndrome (thrombosis of the hepatic vein, causing venous infarction of much of the liver, ascites/acute liver failure)

Arterial thrombosis
• Transient ischaemic attacks/CVA most commonly – myocardial infection/visceral infarction, etc.

Cutaneous
• livedo reticularis
• vasculitis/vasculitic ulcers

Cardiac
• Libman–Sacks endocarditis

Haematological
• Thrombocytopenia in 40%
• Haemolysis

Obstetric
• History of recurrent spontaneous abortions later in pregnancy (second and third trimester; seen in 15–75% of women)
• Intra-uterine growth retardation

Treatment

Treatment is aimed at preventing thrombotic complications, and can involve:
• aspirin (low dose, 75 mg) in milder cases
• warfarin in more severe cases
Patients should avoid the contraceptive pill, keep coronary risk factors low and stop smoking.

PUZZLE 21   SYSTEMIC SCLEROSIS

Systemic sclerosis is a chronic multisystem disorder that causes inflammation, fibrosis and vascular damage to the skin and internal organs. The crossword below contains clinical features associated with this disease. Can you complete it? We have kindly done two for you!

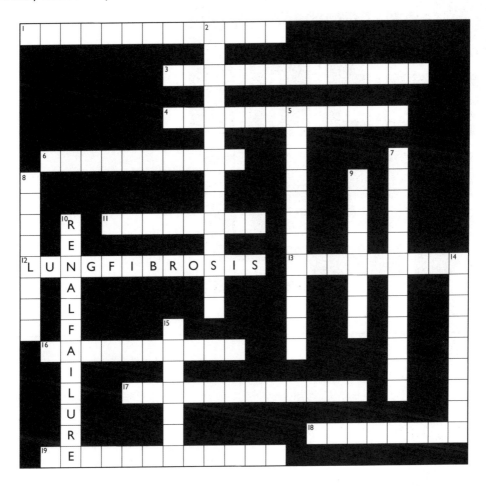

Across

1. Little Malcolm's belly muscles and/or (brief) physical training add up to a particular charge (GI system, 13)

3. Not light-fingered, but more tight-fisted! (Skin of hands, 13)

4. Criminal's start ends in a bung (GI symptom, 12)

6. East-end fireplace on a galari perhaps? (Joints, 10)

11. May be a pain in the arse after football? (Musculoskeletal, 8)

12. It looks like ground glass (4,8)

13. Little Diana starts to run? (9)

16. Laconic sis has a skin problem (Skin, 10)

17. Enough to put your blood pressure up! (Circulation, 12)

18. Sort of French fox, but a bit cold (Circulation, 8)

19. Unable to feel emotion after this? (Circulation, 5,7)

Down

2. I communicate briefly with Angela: electroconvulsive therapy in Asia, perhaps? (Skin, 14)

5. Latin for inflammation around the heart (Heart, 12)

7. My heart burns for you! (Gut, 12)

8. Once claimed to be the reason for the dark skin of a famous popstar becoming lighter (Skin, 8)

9. Re-snogs J, perhaps? (Syndrome, 8)

10. Dialysis a day keeps the docs away! (5,7)

14. Starts out like **6 Across** … but sounds like it is correct that the joints are inflamed! (9)

15. Sounds like you are changing shape here (Skin, 7)

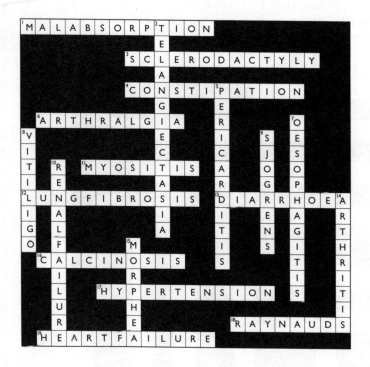

PUZZLE 21   SYSTEMIC SCLEROSIS

Systemic sclerosis is an uncommon (prevalence is 12 per million) multisystem disease of women (80%), characterised by fibrosis of the skin and internal organs.

Limited cutaneous scleroderma begins with tightening of the skin around the fingers (sclerodactyly) and Raynaud's phenomenon; systemic features (eg, disordered oesophageal mobility) may arise later.

With *diffuse cutaneous systemic sclerosis*, Raynaud's starts within 1 year of skin changes and is quickly followed by significant systemic disease (renal, gut, myocardial).

Localised scleroderma (morphea) is characterised by localised skin sclerosis, which rarely, if ever, progresses.

The diagnosis is primarily clinical and management is directed towards providing symptomatic relief; there is no drug treatment to halt disease progression.

Pulmonary and systemic hypertension are major causes of morbidity and mortality. Patients should be monitored closely so that renal and cardiac failure are detected early and treated appropriately. The prognosis depends on the extent of organ involvement. Mean 5- and 10-year survival rates are 60–70% and 40–50%, respectively.

PUZZLE 22   GUESS THE DISTRESS I

This puzzle is a clinical scenario. Read the following passage and then answer the questions.

A 65-year-old lady comes into your surgery. Over the last few weeks she has found it increasingly difficult and painful to rise from a chair and lift herself out of the bath. She has also noticed that her face and neck get sunburned rapidly and that she has developed red plaques over her knuckles. She has suffered from ischaemic heart disease and hypertension for some time, and is currently taking atenolol, bendrofluazide, aspirin and GTN spray.

Questions

1. What is the most likely diagnosis?

2. What other clinical features are characteristic of this condition?

3. What conditions may be associated with this disease?

4. What might investigations reveal?

5. How should the patient be managed?

1. Diagnosis

Weakness and pain of the proximal muscle groups suggest that this lady may be suffering from polymyositis. Since she also has cutaneous involvement (photosensitivity and red plaques over knuckles [Gottron's papules]) she is described as having dermatomyositis.

2. Clinical features

Other clinical features of dermatomyositis include:

- arthritis
- dysphagia
- heliotrope rash over the eyelids (violet)
- periorbital skin rash
- Raynaud's phenomenon

3. Associated conditions

Dermatomyositis is associated with:

- increased incidence of underlying malignancy
- RA
- systemic sclerosis
- SLE

4. Investigations

Investigations may show:

- raised ESR
- raised muscle enzymes (aldolase, creatine phosphokinase)
- anti-Jo-1 auto-antibodies
- characteristic changes on electromyography
- muscle biopsy shows cells infiltrated with macrophages and lymphocytes, muscle cell death and fibrosis

5. Management

- Management is aimed at reducing inflammation using steroid-sparing drugs and corticosteroids.
- Cytotoxic drugs may be required if the disease is severe, fails to respond to corticosteroids or relapses.
- Azathioprine (steroid-sparing drug) is first choice.

Notes

PUZZLE 22 GUESS THE DISTRESS I

PUZZLE 23   SJOGREN'S SYNDROME

Arrange the letters into a cross to produce four clinical features of Sjogren's syndrome. Words can be read forwards, backwards, up and down. One letter has already been put in for you.

One important feature has been missed out. What is it?

TH	RI	YN	IT	S̶	JUN	TI	AUD	KER
HP	RA	AR	EN	IR	CTI	CON	VITI	ATO

Horizontal row (9 boxes): □ □ □ □ [S] □ □ □ □

Vertical column (down from top): □ □ [S] □ □ □ □ □ □

PUZZLE 23   SJOGREN'S SYNDROME

```
                          RA

                          YN

                          AUD

AR   TH   RI   TI   S   IT   IR   HP   EN

                          VITI

                          CTI

                          JUN

                          CON

                          ATO

                          KER
```

In the puzzle are:

Arthritis • Keratoconjunctivitis • Nephritis • Raynaud's

The important clinical feature that has been left out is xerostomia (dry mouth).

PUZZLE 23   SJOGREN'S SYNDROME

Sjögren's syndrome is a chronic auto-immune disorder that usually affects middle-aged women. It is characterised by immunologically mediated destruction and fibrosis of epithelial exocrine glands. It can occur in isolation (primary Sjögren's) or in association with another auto-immune disease (secondary Sjögren's) — typically RA (50% of cases).

The main features are dry eyes (keratoconjunctivitis sicca) and a dry mouth (xerostomia). Labial gland biopsy characteristically shows sialadenitis with lymphocytic infiltration, and a positive Schirmer test is diagnostic (a strip of filter paper is placed inside the lower eyelid — wetting of less than 10 mm in 5 minutes is regarded as positive). ANA antibodies are positive in 70% of cases, and anti-Ro and anti-La in 70% of cases.

Management is aimed at providing symptomatic relief using artificial tears (Hypromellose).

PUZZLE 24 POLYMYALGIA RHEUMATICA

This puzzle is about polymyalgia rheumatica (PMR). When combined with the mystery letter in the centre, the letters in each section of the circle will form four symptoms of PMR. Can you find the missing words and the missing letter?

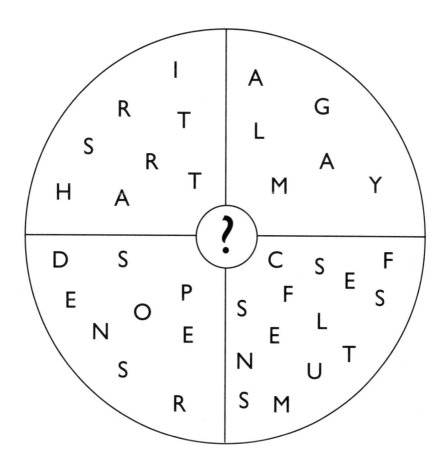

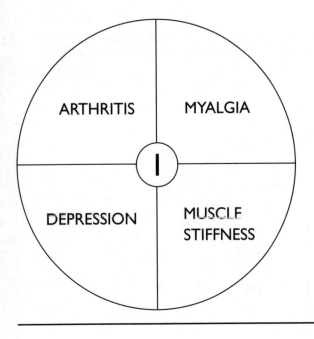

ARTHRITIS | MYALGIA

DEPRESSION | MUSCLE STIFFNESS

PMR is common among the elderly and rare in patients under 50 years of age. Incidence is approximately 1% of the population, and it is associated with HLA-DR4 phenotype.

PMR represents one end of the spectrum that overlaps with temporal arteritis (giant cell arteritis). A total of 15% of patients eventually go on to develop temporal arteritis.

Clinical features

- PMR is characterised by the subacute onset of stiffness and pain in the proximal muscles of the shoulder and the pelvic girdle.
- Patients usually complain of finding it difficult to rise from a chair and get out of the bath.
- Constitutional symptoms include malaise, fever, weight loss and anorexia.
- In patients with co-existent temporal arteritis (see Puzzle 25), there is a localised headache, temporal artery tenderness (sore to brush hair) and loss of temporal artery pulsation.
- Synovitis and bursitis may occur.

Investigations

Very high ESR (may be greater than 100 mm/hour) is characteristic. CRP is also elevated and FBC shows anaemia.

Muscle biopsy shows immune deposition around the fascicles, but no cell infiltration. This is in contrast to polymyositis, where myofibrils are infiltrated with macrophages and lymphocytes (see Puzzle 22). The complexes appear to generate mediators, which cause pain and oedema.

Treatment

- Management is aimed at reducing the inflammation using prednisolone. The dose is altered according to symptoms/ESR and CRP.
- Start 7.5–10 mg of prednisolone. If the symptoms are controlled then reduce by about 1 mg each month. Higher doses and longer treatment are required in those with temporal arteritis. Symptoms usually respond very quickly (within days).

Prognosis

The relapse rate is approximately 25–50%.

PUZZLE 25 GIANT CELL ARTERITIS

The eggs contain symptoms of, or words associated with, giant cell arteritis (GCA). Unscramble the anagram in egg 1 to solve its clue. There will be one extra letter you don't use, which you have to take over to egg 2 to solve that clue, and so on. You will be left with an extra letter after solving the final egg. What is it?

Clues

1. Common presentation (8)

2. Tenderness of this artery may be felt when combing hair (8)

3. "It was like a curtain coming down" (9,5)

4. Can be caused by complete occlusion of the retinal artery (9)

5. Chewing may cause pain in the jaw because of ___ (12)

6. Complication of vertebrobasilar and sometimes carotid involvement (6)

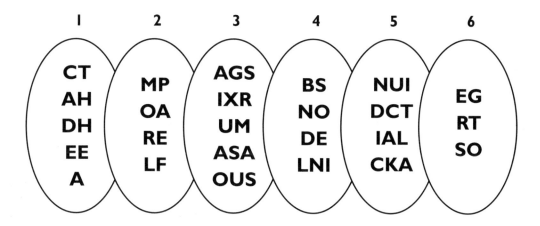

1	2	3	4	5	6
CT AH DH EE A	MP OA RE LF	AGS IXR UM ASA OUS	BS NO DE LNI	NUI DCT IAL CKA	EG RT SO

Investigations

Use arrows to show whether the values for the following blood tests are characteristically increased (↑), normal (↔) or decreased (↓) in GCA:

• Akaline phosphatase
• CRP
• ESR
• Hb
• Platelets

PUZZLE 25 GIANT CELL ARTERITIS

Clinical features

Egg 1: HEADACHE, odd letter = T

Egg 2: TEMPORAL, odd letter = F

Egg 3: AMAUROSIS FUGAX, odd letter = S

Egg 4: BLINDNESS, odd letter = O

Egg 5: CLAUDICATION, odd letter = K

Egg 6: STROKE, left over letter = G

Investigations

• Akaline phosphatase ↑

• CRP ↑

• ESR ↑↑

• Hb ↓

• Platelets ↑

GCA is a systemic disease of unknown aetiology that is characterised by inflammation of medium and large arteries (such as the temporal artery). It usually affects those over 50 years of age, and is relatively common among the elderly (prevalence: 3–5/1,000). GCA is associated with polymyalgia rheumatica (see Puzzle 24) in 25% of people.

It can present in a variety of ways:

- amaurosis fugax/sudden blindness/stroke – visual disturbance occurs in up to 15% of patients
- claudication – patients may get jaw claudication; 15% develop arm claudication
- headache
- scalp tenderness from temporal arteritis
- systemic symptoms are common and include fevers and myalgia

Investigations

ESR is usually markedly raised (often > 100 mm/h) and FBC shows anaemia.

A temporal artery biopsy should be taken. Treatment must be started as soon as the diagnosis is suspected and should not be delayed to wait for the biopsy. The inflammatory changes may not affect the entire length of the artery and skip lesions are common, so a negative biopsy cannot rule out the diagnosis.

Treatment

- If GCA is suspected then high-dose prednisolone (60 mg/day at first) should be given immediately to avoid sudden blindness.
- Treatment should be continued for many months and steroids should be reduced slowly.
- The dose should only be reduced when all symptoms are controlled and the ESR has fallen.

Prognosis

The disease typically lasts for 2 years, followed by complete remission. Unpredictable relapses can occur.

PUZZLE 25 GIANT CELL ARTERITIS

PUZZLE 26   POLYARTERITIS NODOSA

Polyarteritis nodosa (PAN) is a necrotising vasculitis that causes aneurysms of medium-sized arteries. The clinical picture is often highly varied. Non-specific signs and symptoms are characteristic of PAN, with specific features reflecting the site and level of involvement of particular vessels.

Can you fit these blocks together to find seven possible features of PAN? If you are correct, reading down you ought to find the place where two lovers met…

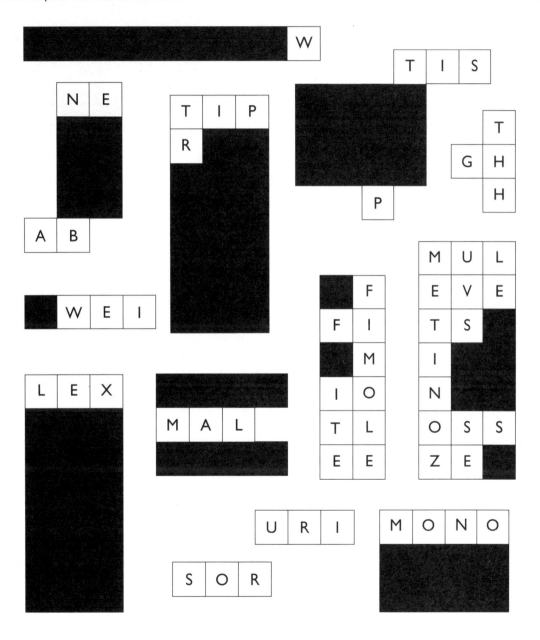

M	O	N	O	N	E	U	R	I	T	I	S	M	U	L	T	I	P	L	E	X
									F	E	V	E	R							
								F	I	T	S									
								M	I											
M	A	L	A	B	S	O	R	P	T	I	O	N								
			W	E	I	G	H	T	L	O	S	S								
			W	H	E	E	Z	E												

In the puzzle are:

Fever • Fits • Malabsorption • MI • Mononeuritis multiplex •
Weight loss • Wheeze

They MET IN OZ!

PUZZLE 26   POLYARTERITIS NODOSA

PAN is a necrotising vasculitis of medium and small arteries
that causes microaneurysm formation, thrombosis and
infarction. It predominantly occurs in middle-aged men.
Many systems of the body are affected.

- Joint pain is associated with general malaise.
- Skin rashes, gut ulceration, gastrointestinal bleeding
  (70%) and renal involvement (haematuria, hypertension,
  proteinuria, renal failure: 75%) are common.
- The lungs can also be involved: when asthma and
  eosinophilia are present, this is known as Churg–Strauss
  syndrome.
- The heart is affected in 80% of patients (coronary arteritis
  with myocardial infarction: pericarditis, heart failure).
- Neuropathies, hemiplegia and fits can occur from cerebral
  involvement.
- WCC is raised (whereas in SLE it is low), as are CRP and
  ESR.
- Raynaud's phenomenon and peripheral neuropathies are
  common.
- On top of all this are malaise, fever and weight loss!

Diagnosis

Diagnosis is largely clinical, but is supported by histological
investigations and renal or mesenteric angiography (usually
show microaneurysms).

ANCA is usually negative. Sometimes PAN is associated with
hepatitis surface antigen; the significance of this is unclear, but
it may be involved in the pathogenesis.

Treatment

- Long-term remission can be achieved using
  corticosteroids and cytotoxic drugs.
- Hypertension is a major cause of mortality and should be
  treated meticulously.

Prognosis

The 5-year survival for untreated PAN is 13%. Death
is commonly due to renal and intestinal and
cardiovascular complications. Unless chronic renal
failure develops, which is uncommon, a normal life span
is expected.

PUZZLE 27   GUESS THE DISTRESS II

This puzzle is a clinical scenario. Read the passage and then answer the questions that follow.

A 76-year-old gentleman comes to your practice with a hot, swollen, painful ankle. He says that the pain started a few days ago, but has now become unbearable. He has also felt quite feverish and cut his knee earlier in the week whilst gardening. He was diagnosed with diabetes mellitus 20 years ago, suffers from hypertension and has a cataract in his left eye. He is currently taking metformin, bendrofluazide and atenolol. He consumes 25 units of alcohol per week.

Questions

1. What is the most likely diagnosis?

2. What is the most likely cause? What is the most common cause of this disease in different age groups?

3. How should he be investigated?

4. How should he be managed?

1. Diagnosis

This is a classic case of septic arthritis. Although cuts/ evidence of a source of infection may be known, this is not always the case. Remember, too, that any source does not have to directly involve the joint (ie, one can cut a thumb and through haematogenous spread of infection develop septic arthritis of a knee).

2. Cause

Septic arthritis can be caused by a number of micro-organisms, the most common of which is *Staphylococcus aureus*. Different micro-organisms tend to be responsible for causing septic arthritis in different age groups.

Bacteria	Group typically affected and comment
Staph. aureus, *Staph. pyogenes*	Adults
Haemophilus influenzae	Children under 6 years
Neisseria gonorrhoea	Young adults
Escherichia coli	Elderly, immunocompromised, intravenous drug users
Mycoplasma tuberculosis	Affects 1% of patients with TB, spine typically affected
Salmonella spp.	Patients with sickle cell anaemia

Odd bacteria can also be involved: thus, evidence of venereal infection may suggest reactive arthritis (see Puzzle 18), but gonococcus can cause both genital infection and spread to the knee joint.

3. Investigation

Septic arthritis is a medical emergency as joint destruction can occur rapidly.

You MUST NOT delay investigation and treatment – HOURS MATTER.

- Joint aspiration. This is the most important diagnostic test. The synovial fluid is purulent, containing >50,000 $\times 10^6$/L leucocytes (90% neutrophils). Gram stain and culture should identify the causative bacterium.
- FBC
- Blood cultures
- Radiographs play little part in diagnosing septic arthritis as it takes some time for joint changes to occur.

4. Management

- This patient should be sent to A&E and treated IMMEDIATELY.
- The joint should be rested and immobilised.
- Broad spectrum antibiotics (flucloxacillin 1 g every 6 hours and benzylpenicillin 1.2 g every 4 hours) should be given until culture sensitivities are known. Antibiotics should be given intravenously for the first 2 weeks, followed by oral antibiotics for 2 weeks.
- Joint aspiration and irrigation with saline may be helpful and must be considered urgently.
- If in the presence of a joint replacement, the prosthetic joint must be immediately removed.

_____

_____

_____

_____

_____

_____

_____

PUZZLE 28   RHEUMATIC FEVER

Join-the-dots to find two images. Why do these represent rheumatic fever so well?

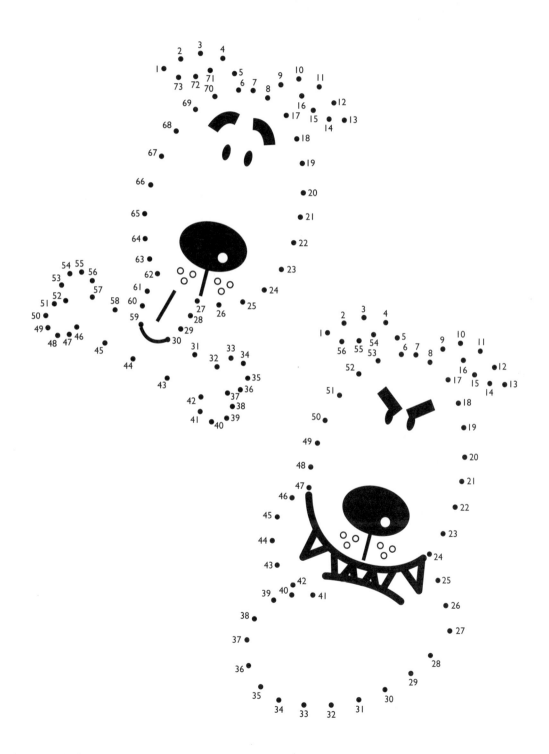

PUZZLE 28   RHEUMATIC FEVER

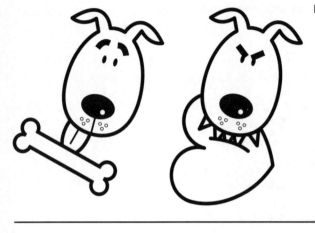

Rheumatic fever 'licks the joints, but bites the heart.'

Rheumatic fever occurs after an infection (often 1–5 weeks after a sore throat) with a group A beta-haemolytic streptococcus. Most cases are in the 6-to 15-year age group.

Auto-antibodies result – these 'lick the joints, but bite the heart'. Larger joints (wrists, knees, elbows and ankles) are most commonly affected. Valvulitis, pericarditis and myocarditis all occur, and can cause early or later valvular stenosis or regurgitation. Carey Coombs murmur is a diastolic mitral valve murmur that is caused by leaflet thickening.

Sydenham's chorea (also known as 'St Vitus' dance') may occur. Rashes (erythema marginatum) and subcutaneous nodules occur.

Diagnosis

Diagnosis is clinical: you need one major and two minor or two major and one minor Duckett Jones criteria (see below), with evidence of recent streptococcal infection (raised antibody levels/positive throat swab/recent scarlet fever).

Major criteria:
- carditis
- chorea
- erythema marginatum
- polyarthritis
- subcutaneous nodules

Minor criteria:
- arthralgia
- fever
- long P-R interval on ECG
- past rheumatic fever
- raised ESR or CRP

Treatment
- Complete bed rest
- NSAIDs
- Benzylpenicillin
- ± Corticosteroids

Treat until ESR is normal, then slowly wean.

Prophylaxis

Prescribe penicillin after an attack to prevent relapse and before dental/other surgery.
Give penicillin for 5 years or until the patient is over 18 years of age.

PUZZLE 28   RHEUMATIC FEVER

PUZZLE 29 GOUT

This puzzle is about gout. From the clues below, work out the words in the maze. The last letter of each word is the first letter of the following word. However, the order of the clues does not reflect the order of the words in the maze. Two letters have been inserted to start you off!

Clues

1. Monosodium urate deposits found in avascular areas, eg, pinna, tendons, joints and eyes – not bean curd! (5)

2. Part of the body first affected in 50% of patients (3,3)

3. Type of drug, used in heart failure, that can precipitate acute attacks (8)

4. Gout occurs when too much urate is made, or its renal … is impaired (9)

5. Drug, other than NSAIDs, used for treating an acute attack (10)

6. Excess consumption of this chemical, in one form, was said to precipitate an attack (7)

7. General advice given to patients to prevent acute attacks, but which may cause them too! (4,6)

8. Analysed under polarised light microscopy to determine the presence of needle-shaped, negatively birefringent urate crystals. May be taken from the knee (8,5)

9. One NSAID used to treat acute episodes (12)

10. A serious renal complication of chronic gout (15)

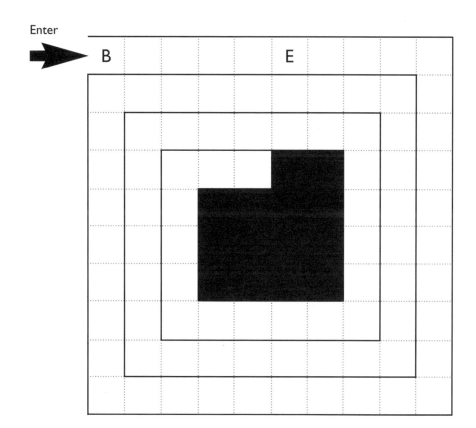

Enter

B   E

PUZZLE 29 GOUT

Enter →

```
  B I G T O E T H A N O
  N E P H R O L I T O L
I U R E T I C O H   L O
C I I O N   L I     O S
A D T ███████ C A   W E
H I E ███████ H S   E W
T U R ███████ I I     E
E L C X E N I C S     I
M F L A I V O N Y     G
O D N I H P O T H G
```

In the puzzle (in order of the clues) are:
Tophi • Big toe • Diuretic • Excretion • Colchicine • Ethanol • Lose weight • Synovial fluid • Indomethacin • Nephrolithiasis

Pathology

Gout is one of the crystal arthropathies (see also pseudogout, Puzzle 30) and usually affects middle-aged men. It is characterised by increased serum urate concentration, recurrent arthritis, aggregated urate deposits (tophi) and renal disease.

Uric acid is formed from the oxidation of purine bases; the kidney excretes 70%, while the rest is lost via the gastrointestinal tract. The causes of gout can be divided into two groups: those that decrease uric acid excretion and those that increase uric acid synthesis.

↓ Uric acid excretion	↓ Uric acid synthesis
Idiopathic (primary)	Idiopathic (primary)
Chronic renal failure	Myelo- and lympho-proliferative disorders
Lead poisoning	Cancer
Drugs (eg, diuretics (especially thiazide), cyclosporin, low-dose aspirin	Excessive alcohol consumption
	Severe psoriasis
Starvation, diabetic ketoacidosis	Lesch–Nyhan syndrome (very rare)

Clinical features

Acutely, gout presents with severe pain, redness and swelling of the affected joint – the first metatarsophalangeal joint of the big toe is most commonly affected. Attacks are due to the deposition of sodium monourate crystals in the joints and may be precipitated by trauma, surgery, starvation, infection, lead poisoning and some drugs.

Cancer patients may be at particular risk, with dehydration and impaired kidney function on the one hand, and massive urate production (cachexia and death of cancer cells with chemotherapy) on the other.

Excessive alcohol consumption was said to be a risk factor – in particular, port. However, in reality, it was lead from the lead crystal in the decanters that caused the gout – so-called 'saturnine gout'.

After repeated attacks, tophi may be found in the pinna of the ear, tendons, joints and the eye.

Diagnosis

Diagnosis is made clinically and on finding negatively birefringent needle-shaped crystals and neutrophils in the synovial fluid of the affected joint. Radiographs show soft-tissue swelling at first; later, periarticular erosions ('punched-out' lesions) are seen in the juxta-articular bone.

Treatment and prognosis

• Acute episodes are treated symptomatically using NSAIDs, eg, indomethacin. If NSAIDs are contraindicated, colchicine is used.
• If the patient is in renal failure then expert help should be sought.
• Attacks may be prevented by losing weight (if indicated, but note that rapid weight loss can cause protein break-down and thus high urate levels), avoiding purine-rich food (offal, oily fish) and avoiding excessive alcohol consumption.
• Long-term drug treatment involves the use of allopurinol or probenecid (these should not be given until 1 month after an attack since they may increase inflammation).
• Unless chronic renal failure develops, which is uncommon, a normal life span is expected.

PUZZLE 30 CALCIUM PYROPHOSPHATE ARTHROPATHY

Unravel the following anagrams to come up with three medical conditions. All cause pyrophosphate arthropathy.

1. PARISH PYRAMID THEORY (19)

2. HI! TOSS MAMA A CHORE (16)

3. OI! THY DISHY ROMP (14)

This anagram tells you the other name for this condition:

4. U PUT EDS GOO (10)

PUZZLE 30 CALCIUM PYROPHOSPHATE ARTHROPATHY

1. HYPERPARATHYROIDISM

2. HAEMACHROMATOSIS

3. HYPOTHYROIDISM

4. PSEUDOGOUT

Calcium pyrophosphate arthropathy (pseudogout) is the most common cause of mono-arthritis (typically of the knee) in elderly women. It is characterised by the deposition of calcium pyrophosphate dihydrate (CPPD) crystals in the articular cartilage and periarticular tissue, causing pain there.

It is often primary, but hyperparathyroidism, haemochromatosis and hypothyroidism are all causes of secondary CPPD disease.

Acute episodes may be triggered by hypophosphataemia and hypomagnesaemia.

Radiographic

- Chondrocalcinosis
- The features of OA:
  – subarticular sclerosis
  – joint space narrowing
  – subchondral cysts
  – osteophytes

Diagnosis

Diagnosis is usually clinical, with radiographic help.

Synovial fluid aspiration:

- pseudogout: CPPD crystals are pleomorphic, rectangular and weakly positively birefringent under polarised light
- gout: urate crystals are needle-shaped and negatively birefringent under polarised light

Check the levels of serum uric acid – these are normal in pseudogout.

Treatment

- Pseudogout is managed by rest, joint aspiration and NSAIDs.
- Intra-articular injections of corticosteroids may also help.

PUZZLE 30 CALCIUM PYROPHOSPHATE ARTHROPATHY

PUZZLE 31 PATTERN OF JOINT INVOLVEMENT

The pattern of joint involvement can give important clues about the underlying condition. A particular pattern of joint involvement links the diseases grouped in the bubbles below. Can you guess what each one is?

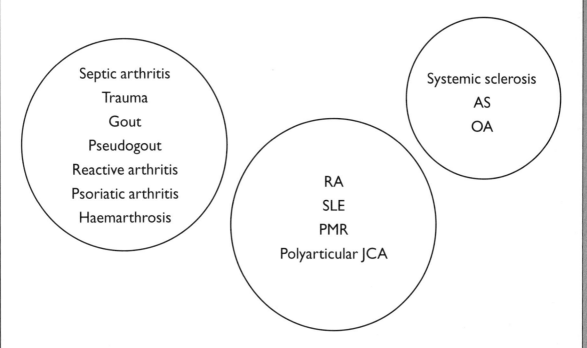

For each group:

- Is the disease symmetrical or asymmetrical?
- Does the disease affect one joint or more than one joint?

PUZZLE 31 PATTERN OF JOINT INVOLVEMENT

Asymmetrical mono/oligo-arthritis

Gout • Haemarthrosis • Pseudogout • Psoriatic arthritis •
Reactive arthritis • Septic arthritis • Trauma

Symmetrical polyarthritis

Polyarticular JCA • PMR • RA • SLE

Asymmetrical polyarthritis

AS • OA • Systemic sclerosis

PUZZLE 32 RHEUMATOLOGICAL RADIOLOGY

Plain radiology often helps with diagnosis, as well as in assessing the severity and progression of a disease. A few very common features of some specific arthritides are found in your patients. Who has which disease, and what is the classical radiological feature?

1. Mavis is waiting for a hip replacement.

2. George has punched-out lesions on X-ray and soft-tissue swelling.

3. David has plantar fascia calcification.

4. One woman has arthritis mutilans on X-ray.

5. The teetotal man has a stiff back.

6. The man with the swollen big toe drinks too much port, and blames this for his disease.

7. The man who smears tar on himself has 'pencil in cup' finger features on X-ray.

8. The man who got drunk with the port-drinker ended up with a venereal disease and arthropathy.

9. One of the women has 'wear and tear' arthritis, and X-rays showing subchondral cysts and osteophytes.

10. Nigel has a 'bamboo spine' on X-ray.

11. Derek met Lucy at the skin clinic, and has pitted nails.

12. Sally has had arthritis since she was a child. She has never met any of the other patients.

Diagnoses
Ankylosing spondylitis • Gout • Osteoarthritis • Psoriatic arthropathy • Reiter's syndrome • Still's disease

Radiological features
Arthritis mutilans • Bamboo spine • Plantar fascia calcification • 'Pencil in cup' finger features on X-ray • 'Punched-out' lesions on X-ray and soft-tissue swelling • Subchondral cysts and osteophytes

Name	Radiological feature	Diagnosis
George	Gout	'Punched-out' lesions on X-ray and soft-tissue swelling
David	Reiter's syndrome	Plantar fascia calcification
Nigel	Ankylosing spondylitis	Bamboo spine
Derek	Psoriatic arthropathy	'Pencil in cup' finger features on X-ray
Mavis	Osteoarthritis	Subchondral cysts and osteophytes
Sally	Still's disease	Arthritis mutilans

All arthritides ultimately leads to narrowing of the joint space, representing loss of cartilage.

RA

Joints affected:
- proximal interphalangeal joints
- second and third metacarpal phalangeal joints
- wrists
- feet

Radiology:
- spindle fingers
- decalcification (osteoporosis)
- subchondral cysts
- joint destruction – this may be mutilating in Still's disease ('arthritis mutilans')

See Puzzles 7 and 8.

Psoriatic arthropathy
- Distal interphalangeal joints with 'pencil-in-cup' appearance.
- Metacarpal phalangeal joints are rarely involved.
- Nail changes are seen.

See Puzzle 17.

Reiter's syndrome
- Calcification around the joint is common.
- Plantar fascia calcification is common (especially at attachment – 'calcaneal spur').

See Puzzle 18.

SLE
- Like rheumatoid, but all the interphalangeal joints are affected

See Puzzle 19.

Ankylosing spondylitis
- Widening of sacroiliac joints then narrowing.
- Calcification of the intervertebral discs and ligaments ('bamboo spine') with kyphosis.

See Puzzle 15.

Osteoarthritis
- Narrowing of the joint spaces (especially knees, hips, spine).
- Osteophytes (outgrowths) at edges of joint.
- Subchondral sclerosis.
- Subchondral cysts.

Gout
- Punched-out lesions.
- Loss of joint space.
- Swollen tissues.

See Puzzle 29.

PUZZLE 32 RHEUMATOLOGICAL RADIOLOGY

PUZZLE 33 ANAGRAMS

Unravel these anagrams to come up with several disease states (and one physiological one). What syndrome can they all cause? Clue: It causes tingling in the hands.

1. PENNY CRAG (9)

2. A! MY IDOL! (7)

3. A CAMEL ORGY (10)

4. YO! MED EXAM! (9)

5. RIOT IT! MARE HIT US HARD (10,9)

6. U GOT (4)

7. IT IS ROOSTER HAT (14)

PUZZLE 33 ANAGRAMS

1. PREGNANCY (physiological)

2. AMYLOID

3. ACROMEGALY

4. MYXOEDEMA

5. RHEUMATOID ARTHRITIS

6. GOUT

7. OSTEOARTHRITIS

The syndrome is:

Carpal tunnel syndrome

PUZZLE 33 CARPAL TUNNEL SYNDROME

Clinical features

Carpal tunnel syndrome is caused by compression of the median nerve as it passes under the flexor retinaculum.

- Burning/tingling/numbness appears in the hand and fingers, and may radiate up the arm as far as the neck.
- The ulnar fingers are often spared, but this is not always the case (some fibres cross over to this territory via the ulnar nerve).
- Symptoms often awaken the patient at night, and are relieved by elevating the arm or submerging the wrist in cold water.
- Muscle weakness may occur – test for weak opposition and abduction of the thumb, and look for thenar wasting.

Diagnosis

Diagnosis is usually made clinically from the history but should be corroborated by nerve conduction studies. Sometimes the tingling can be reproduced by tapping over the flexor retinaculum (Tinel's test; rather nonspecific) or flexing the wrist maximally for 1 minute (Phalen's test; unreliable).

Treatment

Treat the underlying cause. Surgical carpal tunnel decompression may be necessary.

PUZZLE 34   AGE AND SEX!

Most rheumatological diagnoses can be made clinically. As a result, it is extremely important to take a thorough history and perform a complete examination.

About the patient

Age, sex and race are associated with certain rheumatological diseases. Using the diagnoses listed, complete the table below to demonstrate your knowledge of this fact. One disease appears in more than one box.

For a bonus mark, name the disease that Caucasian people are more susceptible to, and another to which Afro-Caribbean people are more prone.

Ankylosing spondylitis • Enteropathic arthropathy • Gout • Osteoarthritis • Polymyalgia rheumatica • Psoriatic arthropathy • RA • Reiter's syndrome • Sjogren's syndrome • SLE

	Predominantly males	Males and females affected equally	Predominantly females
Young			
Middle aged			
Elderly			

	Predominantly males	Males and females affected equally	Predominantly females
Young	Ankylosing spondylitis Reiter's syndrome	Psoriatic arthropathy Enteropathic arthropathy	RA Sjogren's syndrome SLE
Middle aged	Gout		Osteoarthritis RA
Elderly		Polymyalgia rheumatica	

Caucasians are more susceptible to PMR and Afro-Caribbeans are more susceptible to SLE

PUZZLE 35   GOING FOR GOLD – WHAT AM I?

Take a look at this picture. Label as many physical features as you can that may appear in different rheumatological diseases.

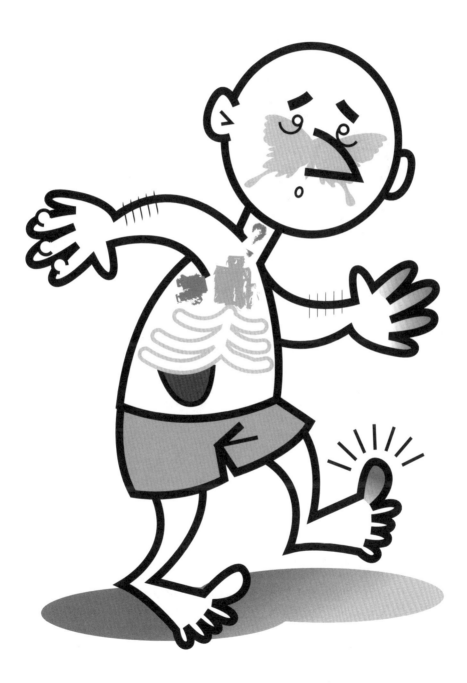

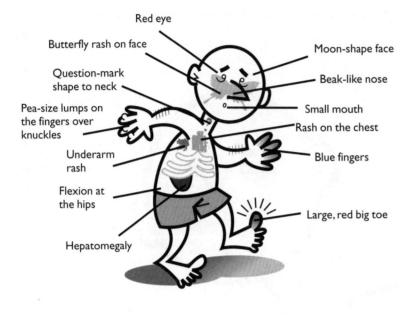

- Red eye
- Butterfly rash on face
- Question-mark shape to neck
- Pea-size lumps on the fingers over knuckles
- Underarm rash
- Flexion at the hips
- Hepatomegaly
- Moon-shape face
- Beak-like nose
- Small mouth
- Rash on the chest
- Blue fingers
- Large, red big toe

PUZZLE 35 GOING FOR GOLD – WHAT AM I?

Here are some tell-tale signs of rheumatological diseases from around the body.

Face

- Beak-like nose – systemic scleroderma
- Butterfly rash – SLE
- Heliotrope rash over eyelids – dermatomyositis
- Moon shape – excess corticosteroids, eg, treatment of RA
- Question-mark shape to neck (hyperextension) – ankylosing spondylitis (AS)
- Red eye – iritis/uveitis caused by RA, seronegative arthropathy
- Small mouth – systemic scleroderma
- Tophi in pinna of ear – gout

Axilla

- Pale-pink macular rash – Still's disease

Chest

- Pleural effusion – SLE
- Rash – SLE, Still's disease, psoriasis, drug reaction, gonococcal arthritis

Abdomen

- Hepatomegaly – Felty's syndrome

Penis

- Circinate balanitis – Reiter's syndrome

Arms

- Nodule over elbow – RA
- Silvery plaque over extensor aspect of arm – psoriasis

Hands

- Ulnar deviation – RA
- Blue digits – Raynaud's phenomenon caused by SLE, systemic sclerosis
- Heberden's nodes over distal interphalangeal joints – osteoarthritis

Legs

- Fixed flexion of hips – AS
- Ulceration – vasculitis
- Large, red big toe – gout

Lymphadenopathy

- Neck, groin, axillae – RA

Notes

Notes

Notes

Notes

INTRODUCTION

Now that you have completed the puzzles (without cheating, we hope!) it's time to get down to business.

Reading the book this way up you will find pertinent text on each of the subject areas covered by the puzzles. Each text highlights the key facts that you need to know, and often offers mnemonics and hints to help your memory along.

When exam time looms, we suggest that you use the book this way up, and read only the 'text' pages. In this way, you will find that you have a complete text (and note) book at your fingertips!